Tea

For

Veterans

Welcome One Home

Reverend Mike Wanner

Table of Contents

Dedication

This book is dedicated to all those who have served to defend the United States of America and their families who have served also, by missing them during their service and some forever. These valiant citizens have given freely in the pursuit of the noble goals specified in the Declaration of Independence and the Constitution of The United States and all the amendments thereto.

I give special recognition to those who have been killed in the service of our country. The citizens now and future citizens of the United States of America will be forever in their debt. May all who have served and their families be blessed in the now and the forever AND SO IT IS!

Special recognition goes also to those injured in the service of our country. The United States of America will be forever in their debt. The injured warriors of our nation have performed well a duty and this writing is offered to help mitigate some of the emotional turmoil that may still reside within those valiant ones. May each of them and their families be blessed in all ways AND SO IT IS!

It is the intent of this work to help Veterans to reclaim their power after their military service is complete.

May All who Read this book be Blessed AND SO IT IS!

Reverend Mike Wanner

Acknowledgements

I would like to acknowledge the support of the following beings:

Ceil Nuyianes is an Earth Angel who started as a student of mine in Reiki and developed into a friend whose book industry expertise helped guide me in many ways.

Mary E Jay who has been an inspiration.

Nancy Russell who was my Integrated Energy Therapy Master Instructor who introduced me to Angel Ariel and the methodology of Heartlinking with the Angels to facilitate the clearing of stuffed emotions and cellular memory.

Stevan Thayer who was my Integrated Energy Therapy Master Instructor Trainer who taught me how to teach others - How to Heal with The Energy of Angels.

My Reiki Masters Rita Hildenbrandt, Hannelore Goodwin, Gary Jirauch, Tom Rigler, Patrick Zigler, Hiroshi Doi, Chiyoko Yamaguchi, Tadao Yamaguchi and especially the founder of Komyo Kai Reiki Reverend Hyakuten Inamoto.

Reverend Ethel Lomardi who taught me the healing power of viewing people as pure light.

Archangels Michael - the Protector, Gabriel - the Communicator, Raphael - the Healer and the legions of Angels that help the healing process for all.

Chapter 1 - Change and Coincidences

Things go together for reasons. Be aware and compare.

Recently

I started the month by going to my local American Legion and Introducing them to my Free Spiritual Healing Book Effort to Help Veterans Healing that I am offering on kindle. The letter that I shared with them is included in a later chapter for your reference but the core of the idea was that I have five free books to offer on Kindle and if you sign up for the notification list, you will be notified when they can be downloaded for free. Free book notification list. - http://VeteransHealing.withRevMike.com .

Recently Also

There was a new healing service offered by the new minister at an Episcopal Church where there has been a great Laying on Of Hands Healing ministry in Reiki which was initiated by two of my Reiki Master Graduates many years ago.

Over the years I had attended many of the Reiki Shares there in order to encourage the continuance of the tradition and the continued spread of Reiki.

I had not been able to attend for quite some time because of two kidney stone operations and eight toe operations and many months of recovery which ended with quite a miracle whereby the IV's that I had been taking for eight years are now history.

Back to the healing service which was quite nice and included collective prayer, prayers for individuals healing, Communion of both bread and wine, anointing with Oil, laying on of hands and sharing.

Before the healing service and subsequent to the Meeting where I shared about the books, I had made a proposal to the American legion to support Veteran Healing. The questions became, How to bring this all together.

Chapter 2 - Alignment of People and Events

This morning as I was doing the dishes, my thoughts turned to the similarities between the churches and the many service organizations like the American Legion, Veterans of Foreign Wars and the Disabled American Veterans. Churches and service organizations could both benefit their organizations and each other and the veterans who need help under the right circumstances.

Creativity could be used in many ways to create an idea with many opportunities to help everybody.

The most exciting idea of it all for me is that cooperation can create good for many more than we are talking about as spinoffs in to the greater community are not only possible, but likely.

The Challenge

Create a Welcome Home Support cooperative effort where there would be three or more participants – A sponsoring Veteran Service Organization, A sponsoring spiritual organization (Church, Synagogue, Mosque or other spiritual Organization) and any veteran who calls ahead or drops in at the Time posted publicly.

Chapter 3 - The Welcome Home

There is great potential here to promote the wellness of:

1. Veterans
2. Churches
3. Service Organizations

The livelihood of all three can be enhanced by taking the effort to embrace Veterans and offer to help them. The secret to success may just be a simple informal meeting where a Service Organization representative and a church representative meet a veteran in an arranged meeting where the priority is simply to chat a bit with no expectations by any of the participants.

I remember well when I came back from Vietnam and went to church with my family. Of course, I had been away for four years and did not know anybody at the particular service I attended. Of course, I expected the same God would be there. I was appalled when there was little good news and a lot of financial reports that I referred to as the Gospel according to the checkbook. I have been to that church seldom since.

Veterans probably do not expect much when they come back. I did not, as Vietnam was not exactly a popular war. It was over twenty years later when someone said "welcome home". And I said "From where" and she said Vietnam. I was surprised and quickly said thanks.

Each Veteran will have different priorities and may or may not be responsive to one of the sponsoring organizations. I would encourage sponsorship teaming that reflects the most likely match that could make a difference in the community.

Churches and Support organizations can, of course, initiate their own programs for the veterans and I would not discourage that. I feel however that there is a built in strength if they do it with a sponsoring partner.

The recommendation is rooted in my belief that the partnership offers veterans:

1. A double layer of resource. With one stop the Veteran can find out about spiritual support and about service organizations.

2. An expedited Welcoming Home that helps them feel welcome and appreciated which can help contain any stressors and jumpstart any needed healing process.

3. The Respect they deserve and the recognition of their service.

4. A support community for the veteran's spouse.

5. Community connectedness for the veteran's family.

The recommendation is rooted in the expectation that sponsors would have

1. An opportunity for sponsoring organizations to be referenced in the newsletter/media/programs of their partner sponsor.

2. An opportunity to have multiple partnerships. Perhaps one service organizations could be aligned with multiple spiritual denominations.

3. Immediate name exposure for the sponsors with the partner sponsor's group.

4. Immediate networking exposure as a participant in the Veterans effort. This may seem a small thing but over time it could make a real difference to the sponsor.

5. A conversation starter where veterans who might never know of the sponsor are invited in to learn about them.

6. A sharing of expertize that can better serve the Veterans.

7. An outreach to the families of Veterans that declares that the sponsor cares about the Veterans.

8. Exposure of the sponsor's programs to the veterans, the veteran's families, the veteran's circle of influence and the partner sponsor's circle of influence.

9. Sponsors may delegate members to participate and get involved so that both the meeting burden and ownership is shared.

The churches and service organization should be prepared to develop the message and resources that they wish to share. Whether there are veterans on day one or not, Sponsors may use the designated time to plan the future format of their events, to pray for veterans or present military or other appropriate tasks.

Prayers can be said each time to further bless the space of the meeting and help form a more inviting venue.

The success of the meetings should include awareness of the needs of the sponsors. Each sponsor would be wise to listen and ask about the needs of their partner sponsors so that the benefit to all can be optimized.

Listening will be a key component to the success of understanding the new needs of veterans. Please know that the historical answer from the war that the service organizations delegates served in may not meet the needs of different theater veterans. Returning Veterans may have new problems and experiences and yesterday's answers may not be the tools that are needed today.

Service organizations have traditions that have been created from the experience of their membership and it may be a big challenge to help with each new war category and it's variables that will only be fully understood once it's veterans start to speak up. That can create a delay which serves not anyone but understanding service organizations can dig in to help.

Churches will also be challenged to find the right prayers, tools, ideas and suggestions that can help the veterans find peace at the earliest possible time.

Chapter 4 - Time for Tea

Conversations about Understanding and Moving Forward

In both English and Japanese traditions, there is great emphasis about Tea or High Tea or the Tea Ceremony or the Tea Rituals.

As I pondered the bridge that is needed to bring Veterans, Service Organizations and Churches together, Tea became a clear potential answer as it conveys the meaning of recognition and respect that sponsors wish to convey to the veterans.

 Scheduling of tea can be simple, inexpensive and productive for both Churches and Service organization. It can be scheduled as often as it seems practical in a given community.

It opens the communication to a new organization of organizations within the community and helps to increase the awareness of all participants and the community members of the cooperating organizations.

Chapter 5 - Organization

To offer Tea, It would be important to have both the spiritual connection and service organization connection. Churches and Service organizations of all kinds would be encouraged to connect with each other so that Tea would have a sponsoring Church/Synagogue/Mosque and a sponsoring Service Organization (i.e. American Legion, Veterans of Foreign Wars, Disabled American Veterans, etc.)

The invited veterans could have understanding listeners from both the service organization and church communities. It could be just the right size first step to safely interact with others.

The Duties of sponsors would include the avoidance of efforts to recruit membership. The support of the veterans would be the only goal. Each supporting organization should understand that supporting the community healing of veterans may well have a desired membership boost over time but recruitment is inappropriate until joining up is the idea of the candidates.

Listening, coaching and mentoring skills can serve sponsors well. Encouraging veterans to talk about anything that interests them can be helpful but an overly precise questioning can cause a level of pushback that can sidetrack the level of trust.

Avoidance of political and religious discussion would be wise to increase the likelihood of the veterans comfort. Job opportunities and educational opportunities may be well received.

Chapter 6 - Sites & Networking

Each sponsor organization will have an interest in receiving some exposure for their participation. It would be wise to discuss dates and locations in advance so that there are no problems created by misunderstandings that could later jeopardize the cooperation of key personnel.

Perhaps, the venue could rotate monthly or quarterly as agreed. Notices within each organization should freely reference the cooperating sponsors name, venue locations, contact person names and contact details (i.e. Phone numbers, e-mail addresses etc.)

It is important that sponsors directly and politely discuss any sensitivities that there may be about a venue that may be of a different faith than their own. It may even make sense for some overlapping networking where one service organization may have different religious connectivity from month to month on some rotation as determined by the mix and interests within a given community.

The optimal plan may contain multiple neighboring organization details so optimal comfort and/or spiritual affiliation could add to the Veteran's options and connectedness.

Chapter 7 - What Happens If No One Comes to Tea?

Sponsors should understand that it may take some time for Candidates to show up. It may be a good idea to agree in advance to a prayer ritual or agenda in case someone does not show up. Helping each unsupported veteran is a huge success for the restoration of their life and the furtherance of peace on earth.

Whether or not anyone shows up the first couple of times, prayers can be said for the country, veteran community, those still in uniform and especially for the families of all those who have ever served. The opportunity of the scheduled event can be used as the creation of sacred space for future meetings.

The scheduling of Tea can be thought of as the first step of the process. If you were building a structure, you would pour the foundation and then you build up from there.

Scheduling the Tea every month on the organizational schedules declares your openness to welcoming Veterans. Your members can then tell their family and friends of the organizations program. Having partners also helps to get the word out about the program and the existence of your organization.

Chapter 8 - Sensitivity

Sponsors would be wise to hyper-activate their listening skills and recognize words that are applied by veterans to themselves and then determine what words may be soothing and what words should be avoided.

The veteran's perspectives of words and situations may be different than a civilian. Listening about tags and labels will also prove insightful to sponsors.

While the focus is on the veteran, spouses and families can offer a lot of help to the sponsors. Not all veterans will want to go there in conversation so patience and responsiveness Is very helpful.

When opportunity to chat about family is welcome, it may feel appropriate to bring out your pictures and share on a personal level.

Chapter 9 - Things for Sponsors to Discuss

The structure of Tea:

1. Rituals
2. Denomination etiquette
3. Warm welcome
4. Casual mood
5. Pace as Invitational and Incremental but not pushy
6. An expectation of acceptance but not a need for it
7. Pauses for perspective
8. Coaching language may prove helpful
9. Asking about personal goals may prove helpful
10. Ask about comfort levels:
    a) Changing Expectations
    b) Topic choices
    c) Veterans in Charge
    d) The partnership pace
    e) Reiki for Reverends and others
    f) Blessing Medication
    g) PR & TV as agreed and appropriate
    h) Video Developing
    i) Healing
    j) The pieces of Your personal Power
    k) Permission to be Videoed, taped etc.?
    l) Progression-
        i. People from a Church - Minister, Deacon, Members, Congregants, Veterans Families
        ii. The People from a Service Organization - Leader, / Member
11. Any other matters of importance for success

Chapter 10 - Free Spiritual Healing Book Effort to Help Veterans

Rev. Mike Wanner
7340 Rising Sun Ave.
Philadelphia, PA 19111 USA
215-342-1270
E-mail: mikewann@voicenet.com

Re: Free Spiritual Healing Book Effort to Help Veterans

I invite you to join the Veterans Healing Book Notification List at http://VeteransHealing.withRevMike.com

I wrote about Trauma Healing Options. The first book is titled Trauma Healing Options For VA Hospitals: Help for Veterans to Own Their Significance and Their Future.

That book was followed with four others that are of the Do It Yourself Variety. The First of those books is called Trauma Healing Action Steps for Veterans: Help To Start Healing and the second is called Trauma Healing Action Steps for Veterans: Empowerment and the third is called Trauma Healing Action Steps for Veterans: Forgiveness.

The fourth is called Trauma Healing Action Steps for Veterans: Thought Freedom.

The VA has a lot of traditional care available for Veterans to help us heal. While the media reports problems and scandals, there is a tremendous force of professionals dedicated to helping us vets and these folks can do a lot for us. I am personally very grateful for the care that I have received at the Philadelphia VA Medical Center.

The books that I have written are to be turned in to a Free spiritual non-denominational support system for Veterans. I will use the Kindle promotional system to giveaway copies of the books each month. Kindle will allow an author to do a free five day giveaway every 90 days and I have five books so I can give one away every thirty days and two some months.

No Kindle is required to download the books. Amazon.com has a free application that offers "Kindle for PC" software and "Kindle for Mac" software where you can download the appropriate application and then download the books when they are offered.

Things to Know

These books are not a substitute for Professional services. On the contrary, they are intended to help veterans to find resources and people who they can help and those who might help them.

Veterans have been trained many ways and while they may temporarily be in an overwhelm type of situation from time to time, there is a huge likelihood that they can help many others as they themselves reground their energies and realign their efforts.

To sign up for the notification list, go to http://VeteransHealing.withRevMike.com

I would appreciate any evaluations or suggestions you might have about spreading the word about these books. I also would be happy to help organize any of the programs that are mentioned in the first book.

Frequently Asked Questions

Are the books available at others times?

Yes, the books are always available on Kindle but I can only use the system to distribute them FREE once a month.

Are the Books available in Print?

Yes, the books are available in print through Amazon.com and other book sellers.

Chapter 11 - Conclusion

Many times I hear from folks that they don't know what they are supposed to do with their life and they fret about it.

In my experience, the messages from our God are there but sometimes they are difficult to hear because our senses are hyper-stimulated. If you will just turn off the TV, the computer, the cell phone, the tablet and the newest device you own for a little while, then you can enter the silence and hear the still small voice within.

God loves each of us now and forever regardless of how we have behaved. As you read this, take a moment to say hello to God. If you would like to help veterans, you may cause God to smile.

*

Toastmasters Wanted

Please give speeches about:

1. This Book - Tea For Veterans
2. The Veterans Healing Notification List Sign
   Up Site in Chapter 10.

ReverendMikeWanner.com
Resources List

Distant Healing Sessions –

Physical Healing
http://LetMeHelpYouHeal.withMike.com

Angel Healing
http://AngelHealing.withmike.com/

Books by Rev. Mike at www.Amazon.com–

Veterans Healing Six Pack:
1. *Trauma Healing options for VA Hospitals: Help for Veterans to Own Their Healing and their future.*
2. *Trauma Healing Action Steps for Veterans: Help to Start Healing*
3. *Trauma Healing Action Steps for Veterans: Empowerment*
4. *Trauma Healing Action Steps for Veterans: Forgiveness*
5. *Trauma Healing Action Steps for Veterans: Thought*
   Freedom
6. *Tea For Veterans: Welcome One Home*

Angel Raphael Speaks Volume One: Take Courage!
God Has Healing in Store for You

Angel Raphael Speaks Volume Two: Take Courage!
God Has Healing in Store for You

Reiki Journaling from Japan

Reiki Is Alive: God's Great Gift

Four Parts to Healing

Distant Healing: We Are All Connected

Stress Release Energy Work: How To Cope

Does Reiki Love Heal Cancer?

Group Consciousness

Free Resources

Learn to dump fear at
http://TheGreatAmericanFearDump.withMike.com

Spiritually Prepare for Surgery
http://PrepareForSurgery.withRevMike.com

Angel Scribe messages at
http://www.SpiritualComfortCare.com

Law of Attraction Expert column at
http://www.ReverendMikeWanner.com

Stress Release at
http://www.StressReleaseCoach.com

   Angel Raphael Speaks through Rev. Mike Wanner. I have channeled multiple message sets and they all have to be polished to smooth out my errors and negotiate some words that may be too easily misunderstood. Grammar is not polished as it is too easy to miss the subtlety of the energy flow. To find out the availability of messages and latest updates go to
http://www.spiritualcomfortcare.com/angel-raphael-speaks/

Also "Tell Mike your concerns – If he and I agree there is a broader need, messages may follow. Citizens of all nations invited as long as your write in English. Do not expect him to answer as he is very busy already listening to us." E-mail Mike at
mikewann@voicenet.com.

May All Who Read This Be Blessed
Reverend Mike Wanner

Join the Veterans Healing FREE Kindle Book
Notification List at
http://VeteransHealing.withRevMike.com

Private Channeling

Angel Raphael Speaks is a series of free messages that are channeled through Reverend Mike Wanner for the Highest good and Highest Healing of all concerned.

Many questions arise about Reverend Mike doing private channeling and he does help with that at his site http://AngelHealing.withMike.com

Reverend Mike is available world-wide as a psychic channel, emotional release facilitator, spiritual energy practitioner & teacher, and public speaker. He looks forward to meeting you soon!

Email - mikewann@voicenet.com 215-342-1270
http://AngelHealing.withMike.com

PRIVATE SPIRITUAL READINGS/channelings or Spiritual Healing Sessions: Telephone or in person

Rev. Mike is available for private, one-on-one intuitive sessions with you, his Guide Family, and your Guides. He helps by offering clarity on emotional situations about your life, your purpose, your spirituality, and the release of stuffed emotions and cellular memory.

Connect to the love of your Guides today!

Contact Rev. Mike for an appointment.

Click on this link to go to the page – http://AngelHealing.withMike.com

Sessions available:

Spiritual Readings
Angel Channeling
Distant Reiki Healing
Distant Clearing of Stuffed Emotions
Distant Clearing of Cellular Memory
Distant Clearing of Energy Blockages
Distant Clearing of the Chakras
Mastermind dowsing responses to yes/no direction finding questions.
Customized needs

Rev. Mike is a facilitator of healing. He brings you and the Divine together so that you can align with the Divine and have a great time and a great life. All healing is between you and God, as it should be. Go ahead and start without

Rev. Mike. Visit his prayer site http://www.Create-A-Prayer.com. Take the first step NOW.

Rev. Mike Wanner

Rev. Mike Wanner started his metaphysical and ministerial studies with Reiki in 1993 and has studied seven styles of Reiki in the U.S., Japan, Canada, Denmark and Australia. He is certified to teach. He became certified to teach Integrated Energy Therapy in 1999 and co-taught the first IET class of the new Millennium. Mike began dowsing in 2001.

Ordained as a Metaphysical Minister of the International Metaphysical Ministry and an Interfaith Minister of the Circle of Miracles Ministry, Rev. Mike practices and teaches spiritual energy therapies in the Philadelphia Area.

Rev. Mike holds ministerial degrees from the University of Metaphysics and the University of Sedona. He is a Pastoral Care Associate of Aria – Frankford Hospital. He taught at the National Academy of Massage Therapy and Health Sciences.

Rev. Mike was a faculty member of the Medical Mission Sister's Center for Human Integration's School of Integrated Body/Mind Therapies in Fox Chase, Philadelphia, PA for twelve years.

Rev. Mike is licensed by the teaching of Intuitional Metaphysics to practice Spiritual Healing and Scientific Prayer. Mike is also a Prayer therapist.

Rev. Mike was elected in 2007 to the status of "Fellow of the American Institute of Stress."

In 2008, Rev. Mike became a practitioner of Coincidental Recognition as he incorporated the CoRe system in to his spiritual healing practice.

In 2009, Rev. Mike trademarked a new healing process called Quantum Quatro! Subtle Energy System Support®.

In 2011, Rev. Mike joined the outreach program known as the Health Advantage Group.

In 2012. Rev. Mike became a Certified Professional Coach by The Master Coaching Academy and Joined The Personal Empowerment Group .

Prior to his metaphysical, ministerial and coaching studies, Rev. Mike worked for Sears Roebuck and Co. while in High School and after graduation until he joined the U. S. Air Force in 1965. He returned to Sears from Vietnam in 1969 and stayed until 1978. His final Sears assignment was as an efficiency expert in Methods - Operational Research and Development. He volunteered with Burholme Emergency Medical Services from 1969 and is still a Life Member and Board of Directors Member. He started a private ambulance company in 1975 and worked professionally in the field until 2001 when he devoted his full attention to real estate investing, healing and coaching.